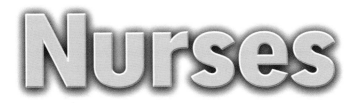

Nurses

by Marlene Targ Brill

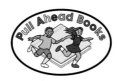

Pull Ahead Books

Lerner Publications Company • Minneapolis

To all the nurses who help us feel better

A hearty thank you to Diane Bader, Wilmette public health
nurse, and Barbara Kennedy, American Nurses Association,
for answering my questions for this book

Text copyright © 2005 by Marlene Targ Brill

Lerner Publications Company
A division of Lerner Publishing Group
241 First Avenue North
Minneapolis, MN 55401 USA

Website address: www.lernerbooks.com

Words in **bold type** are explained in a glossary on page 31.

Library of Congress Cataloging-in-Publication Data

Brill, Marlene Targ.
    Nurses / by Marlene Targ Brill.
        p.   cm. — (Pull ahead books)
    Includes index.
    ISBN: 0–8225–1692–6 (lib. bdg. : alk. paper)
    1. Nursing—Juvenile literature. I.Title. II. Series.
RT61.5.B75 2005
610.73–dc22   2004019585

Manufactured in the United States of America
1 2 3 4 5 6 – JR – 10 09 08 07 06 05

Scratch, scratch!

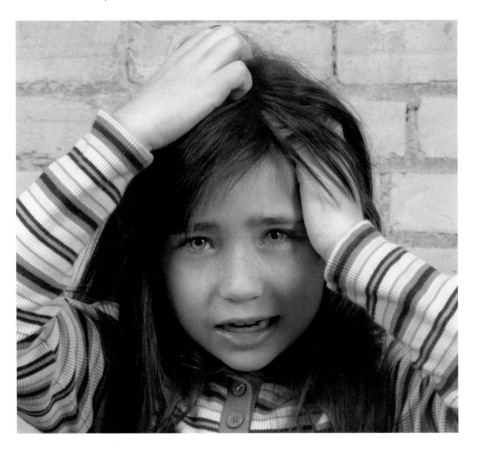

What's on your head?

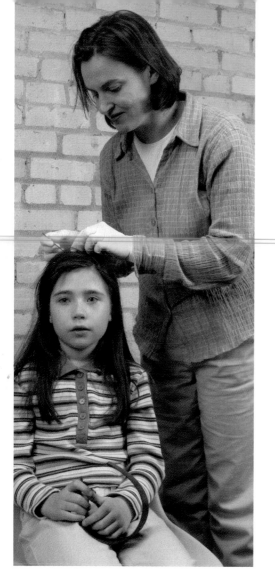

School nurses know. They make sure students are healthy.

School nurses check for itchy head lice.

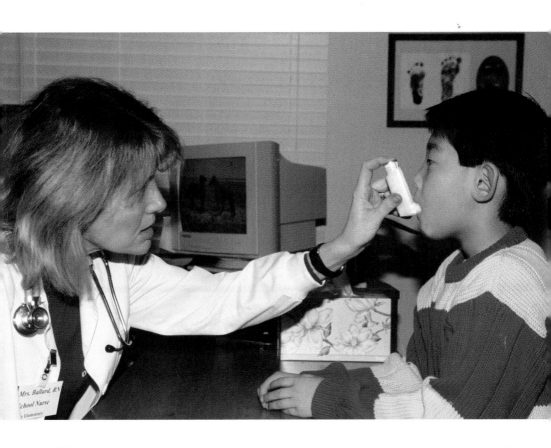

They teach students how to take care of themselves. School nurses help students with special health needs.

School nurses also test how well students see and hear. Where else do nurses work?

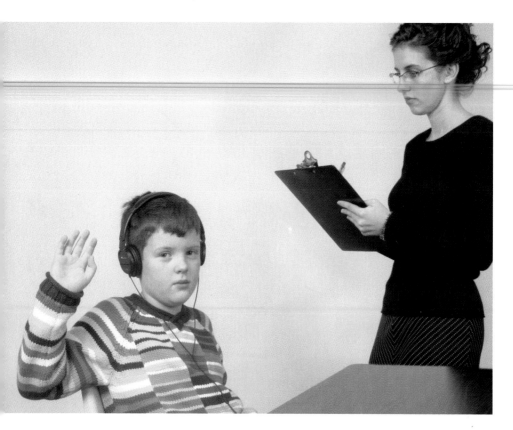

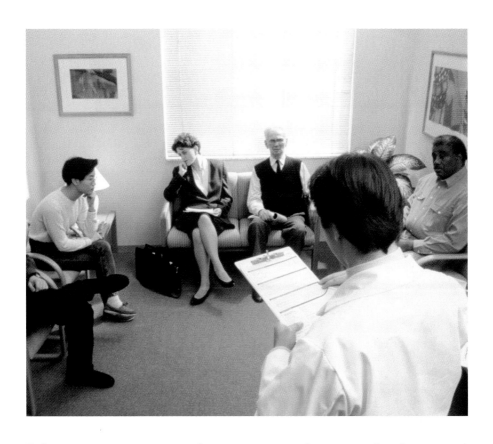

Many nurses take care of people in hospitals or doctors' offices in the **community**.

Some nurses take care of people who cannot leave home. These nurses may visit many days a week.

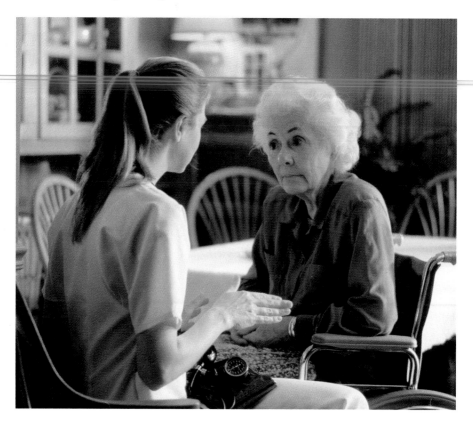

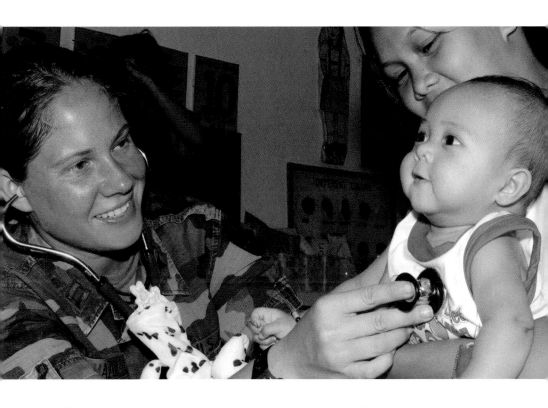

Other nurses join the armed services
and help people around the world.
How do nurses know how to make
people feel better?

Nurses go to nursing school after high school. They learn about giving health care.

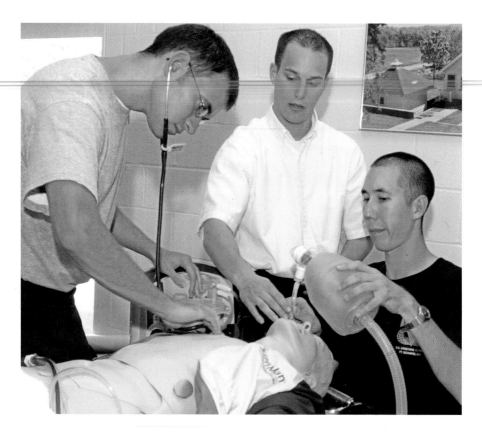

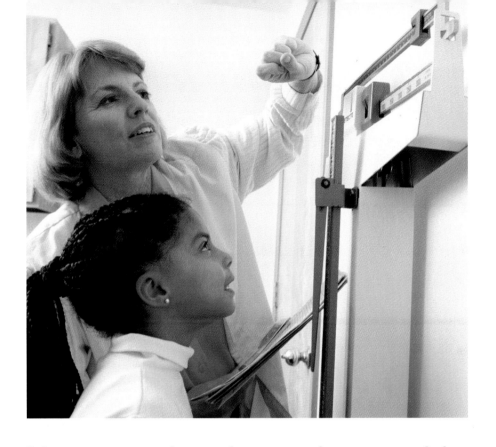

Many nurses learn how to do some of the same things doctors do. Nurses collect information that doctors need. They measure your height and weight.

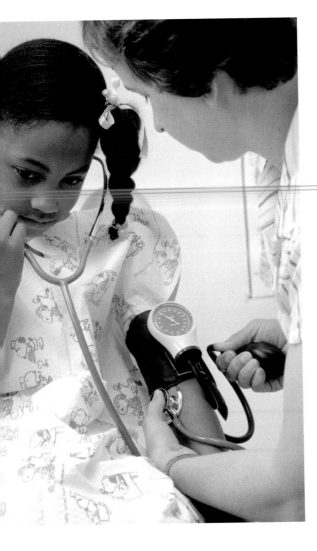

They take your
blood pressure.
Blood pressure
shows nurses
how well your
blood pumps
through your
body.

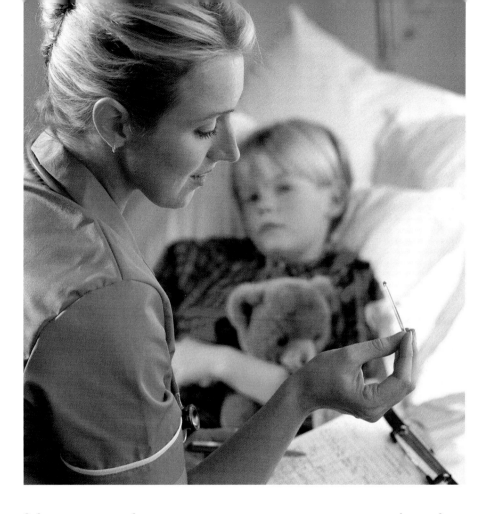

Nurses take your temperature and ask questions about how you feel.

Nurses make **records** of this information. Records help doctors and nurses keep track of your health.

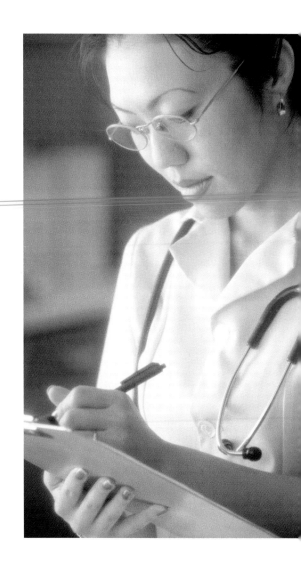

Nurses work closely with doctors to keep you healthy.

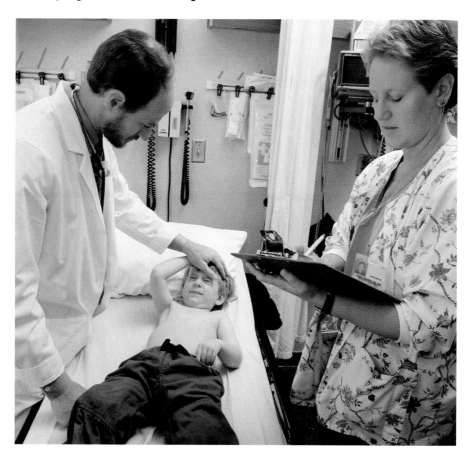

Nurses give **medicines** that doctors order. Medicines are pills or shots that make you feel better.

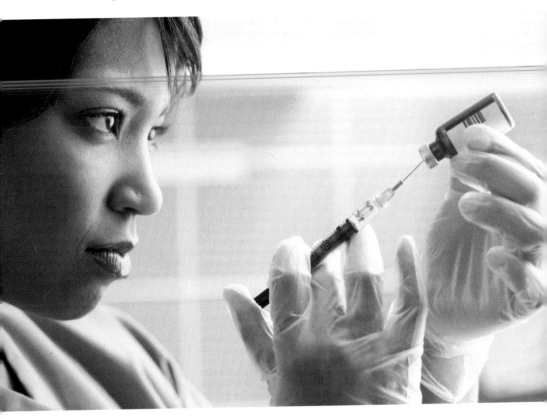

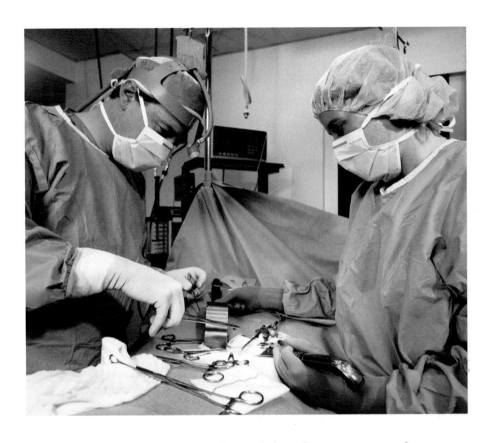

Some nurses work with doctors who **operate.** The doctor cuts into the body to fix something inside.

Other nurses work in the **emergency room.** They take care of people who need help right away.

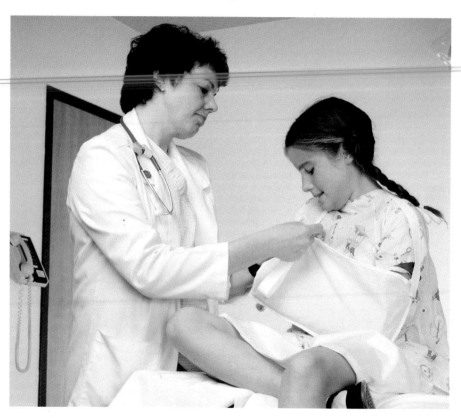

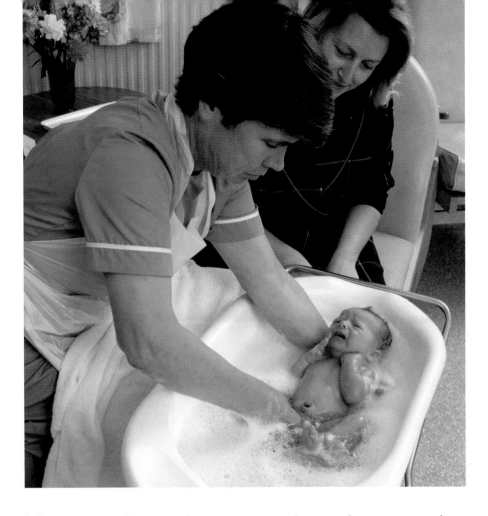

Nurses also take care of mothers and their newborn babies.

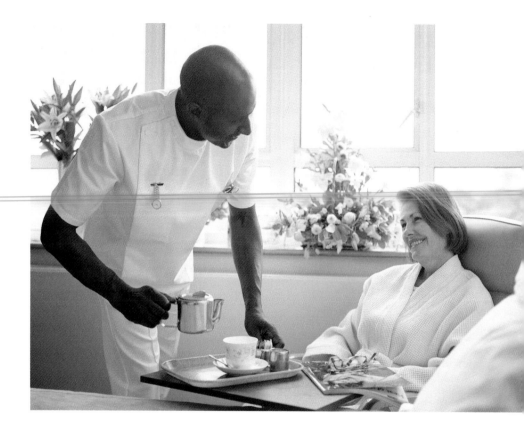

Some nurses give bedside care. They
serve meals to people staying in the
hospital.

They help keep sick people clean
and comfortable.

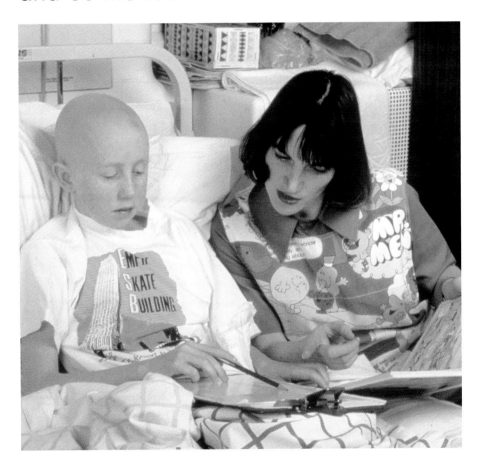

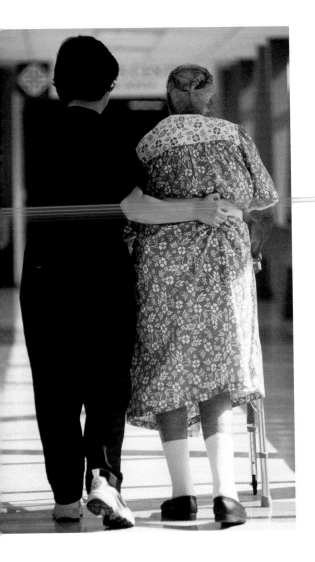

What makes
a good nurse?
Nurses are
helpful and
caring.

They must be strong to lift people who can't help themselves.

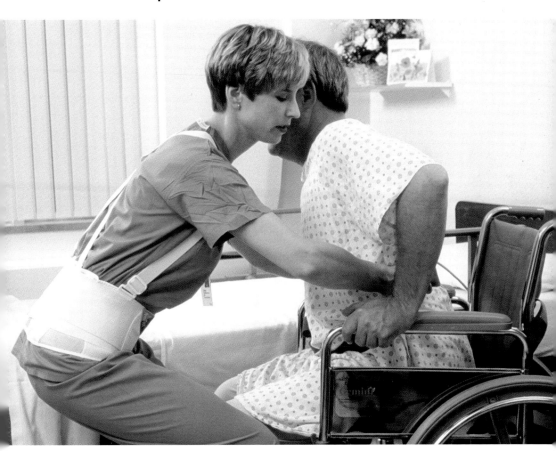

Nurses like science and learning
about the body.

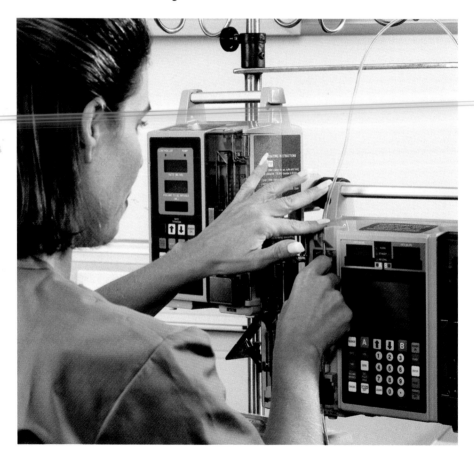

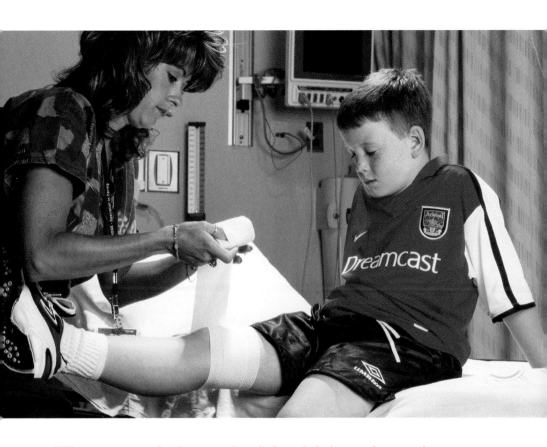

They can't be afraid of blood and broken body parts. They must stay calm during emergencies.

Nurses work hard both days and nights. Why would anyone want to work so hard?

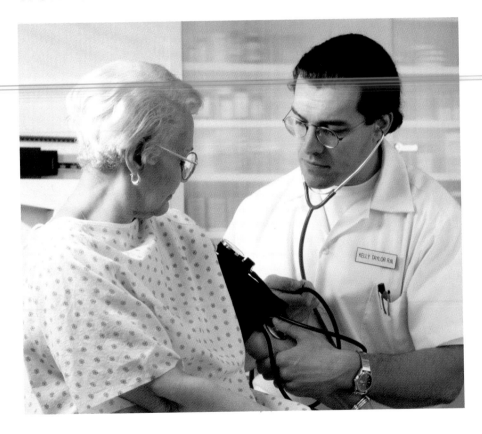

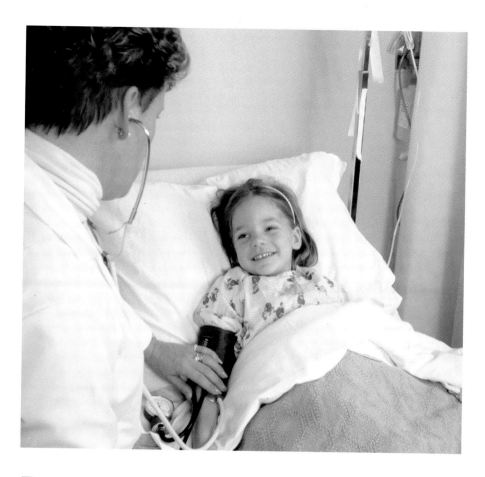

Because nurses feel good about
helping people feel better.

Facts about Nurses

- Nurses can be women or men. About 5 in every 100 nurses are men.

- Most nurses carry out doctors' orders. But some nurses work on their own. They are called nurse practitioners.

- Nursing schools are run by hospitals or colleges. With more schooling, a nurse can oversee more jobs and people.

- Nurses who work in hospitals earn the most money.

- Nursing is one of the fastest-growing community jobs.

Nurses through History

■ The first nurses were slaves in ancient Roman homes. They taught rich Romans how to mix plants into medicines.

■ Florence Nightingale opened the first nursing school in Great Britain in 1860.

■ Dorothea Dix led the first group of U.S. Army nurses during the Civil War (1861–1865). Her work began the Red Cross. This group helps people in need around the world.

■ Early nursing schools refused to let in African Americans. Mary Mahoney became the first black nurse in 1879.

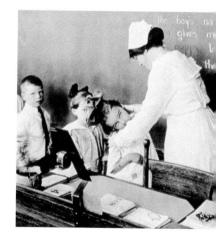

■ May is National Nurses Month.

More about Nurses

Books

Flanagan, Alice K. *Ask Nurse Pfaff, She'll Help You.* New York: Children's Press, 1998.

Ransom, Candice. *Clara Barton.* Minneapolis: Lerner Publications Company, 2003.

Storring, Rod. *A Doctor's Life: A Visual History of Doctors and Nurses through the Ages.* New York: Dutton Children's Books, 1998.

Wohlrabe, Sarah C. *Helping You Heal: A Book about Nurses.* Minneapolis: Picture Window Books, 2003.

Zemlicka, Shannon. *Florence Nightingale.* Minneapolis: Carolrhoda Books, Inc., 2003.

Websites

Future Nurses Kids Club Website
http://www.sc.edu/nursing/KidsClub/KidsClubIndex.html

KidsHealth
http://www.kidshealth.org/kid/

The Nursing Gang
http://www.discovernursing.com/gang/

Way Cool Surgery: Medical Careers
http://www.waycoolsurgery.com/careers/nursing.shtml

Glossary

community: a group of people from one neighborhood, town, or city

emergency room: part of the hospital that gives care right away

medicines: drugs people take to treat illness

operate: what a doctor does to fix a sick part of the body

records: facts written down and kept on file about a person or group

Index

Photo Acknowledgments

The photographs in this book appear courtesy of: © Todd Strand/Independent Picture Service, front cover; © Sam Lund/Independent Picture Service, pp. 3, 4, 6; © Jack Ballard/Visuals Unlimited, p. 5; © Jose Luis Pelaez, Inc./CORBIS, pp. 7, 14, 26; © Gary D. Landsman/CORBIS, p. 8; © James-Denton Wyllie/U.S. Army, p. 9; © AP|Wide World Photos, p. 10; © Tom Stewart/CORBIS, p. 11; © Blair Seitz/Photo Researchers, Inc., p. 12; © Digital Vision Ltd./SuperStock, pp. 13, 20; © Royalty-Free/CORBIS, pp. 15, 17, 18, 24; © JLP/Sylvia Torres/CORBIS, p. 16; © Jennie Woodcock/Reflections Photolibrary/CORBIS, p. 19; © Simon Fraser/Photo Researchers, Inc., p. 21; © ER Productions/CORBIS, p. 22; © Ed Bock/CORBIS, p. 23; © Richard T. Nowitz/CORBIS, p. 25; © Larry Mulvehill/Photo Researchers, Inc., p. 27; © CORBIS, p. 29.